Sea Otter Cove

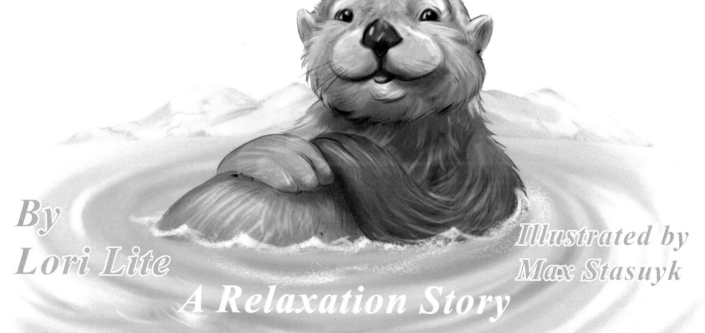

By
Lori Lite

Illustrated by
Max Stasuyk

A Relaxation Story

Congratulations!

Welcome to *Sea Otter Cove*.
It is fun to pretend that you are the sea child or that you are
the sea otter as you imagine your own warm rock to rest on.
Get comfortable, close your eyes and enjoy breathing.

NOTE TO PARENTS: Relaxation breathing works best when the belly rises from the inhale and the belly falls on the exhale. Most of us are not familiar with this feeling of belly movement. The exercise in the story of blowing a feather away is just a way for your child to get their belly moving. Another way that helps children experience their belly moving is to roll onto their side which helps the belly relax. Remember the belly should lift on the inhale during the breathing sequence and fall on the exhale. We do not want to overemphasize or cause stress trying to breathe correctly. Bringing awareness to breathing is already a big step.

(For a variation of this breathing exercise, children can breathe in through their nose and let the air out of their mouths saying ahhh...) Enjoy!

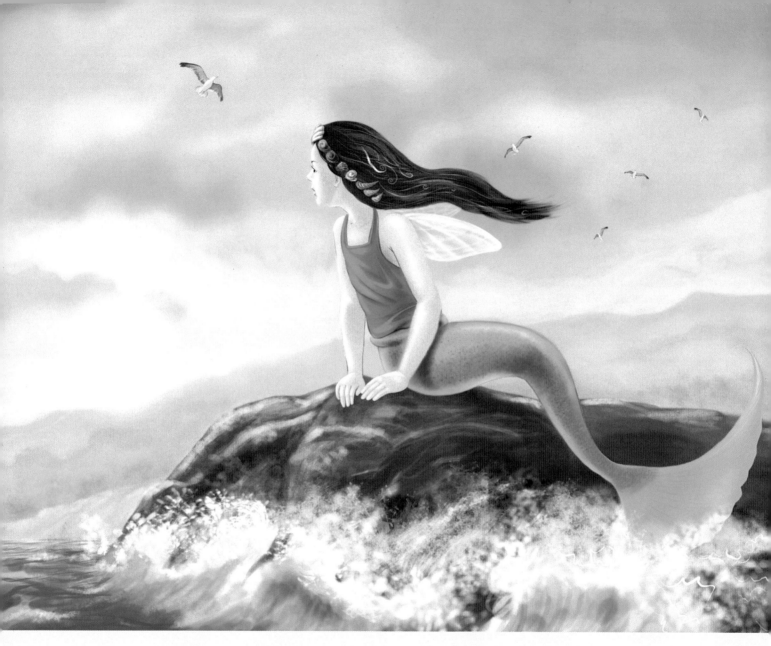

A sea child sat on a large rock in the middle of
a shallow cove surrounded by high cliffs.
This was one of her favorite places to
relax and clear her mind.

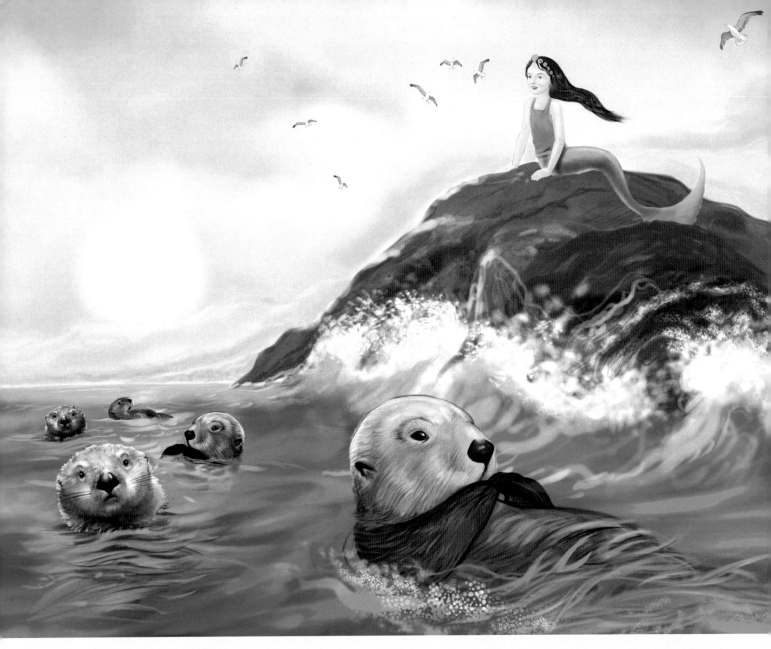

Many sea otters would come to this cove to eat, play, and rest in the kelp beds
that hugged the rock. The sea otters loved to drape the long kelp
over their bodies and drift gently on the waves.
This special place was called Sea Otter Cove.

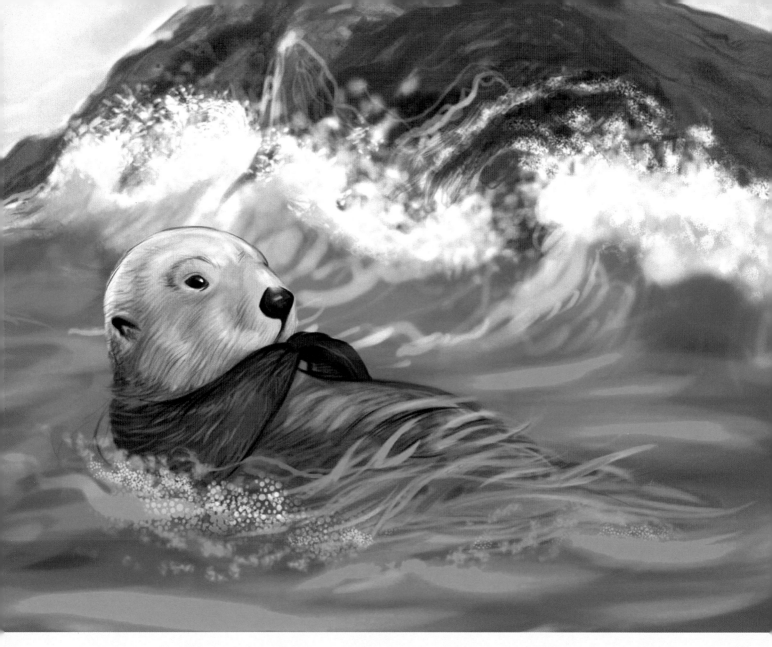

The sea otters liked to share their hideaway with the sea child.
They all knew that this was a great place to rest, relax,
and warm their bodies in the sun.

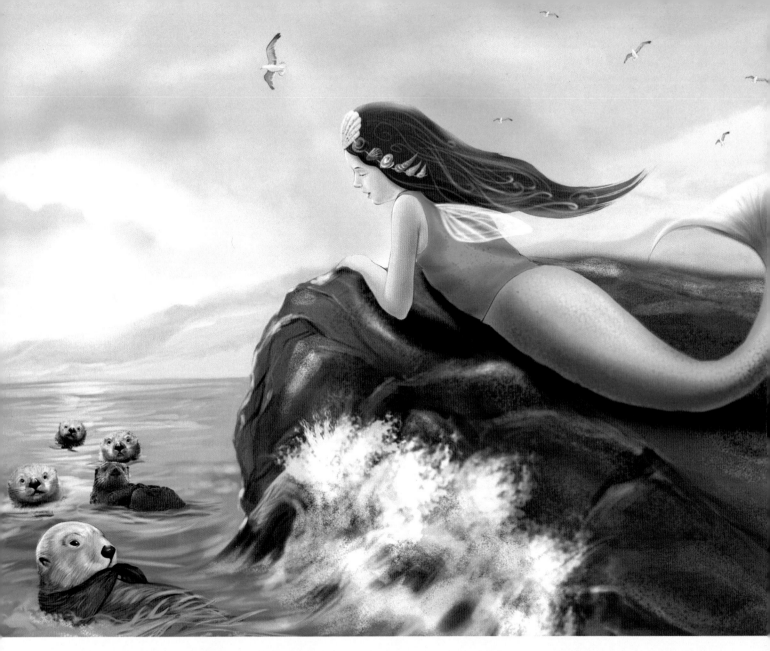

The swirling colors of the rock were perfect for absorbing the sun's pure, white light. The sea child loved how the heat felt as she made herself comfortable. She wiggled her body until she could feel her spine and back relaxing into the rock. She closed her eyes and listened to the sound of the sea otters playing in the waves that splashed against the rock.

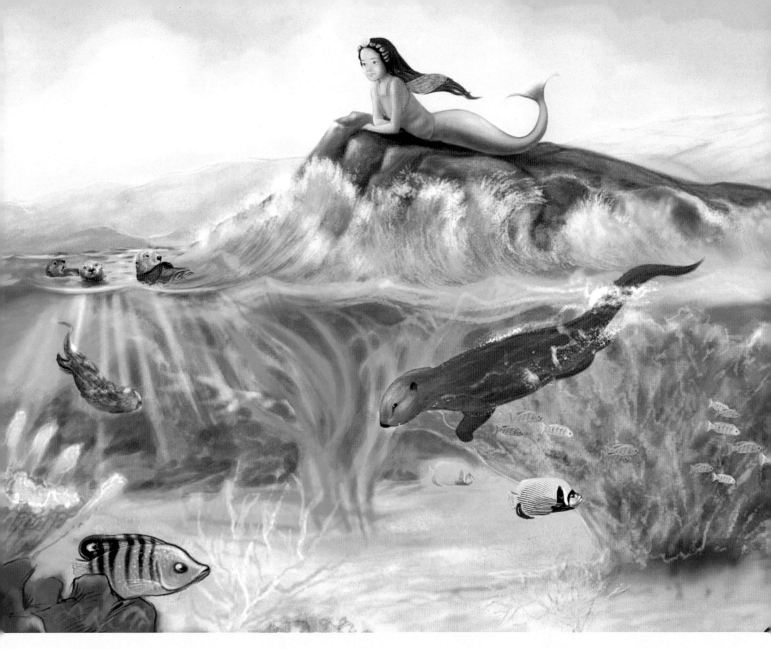

The rock stood strong against the ocean's waves. The sea child imagined that the rock extended down through the ocean and kept going, right through the sand, connecting her to the center of the earth.

She felt safe and anchored.

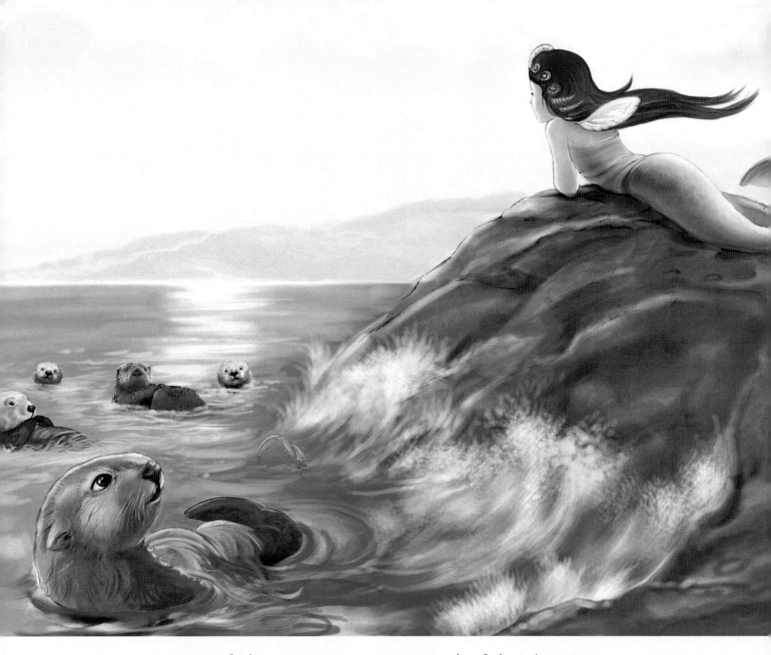

One of the sea otters was very playful and curious.
He liked to hide behind the rock and watch the sea child
whenever she came for a visit.

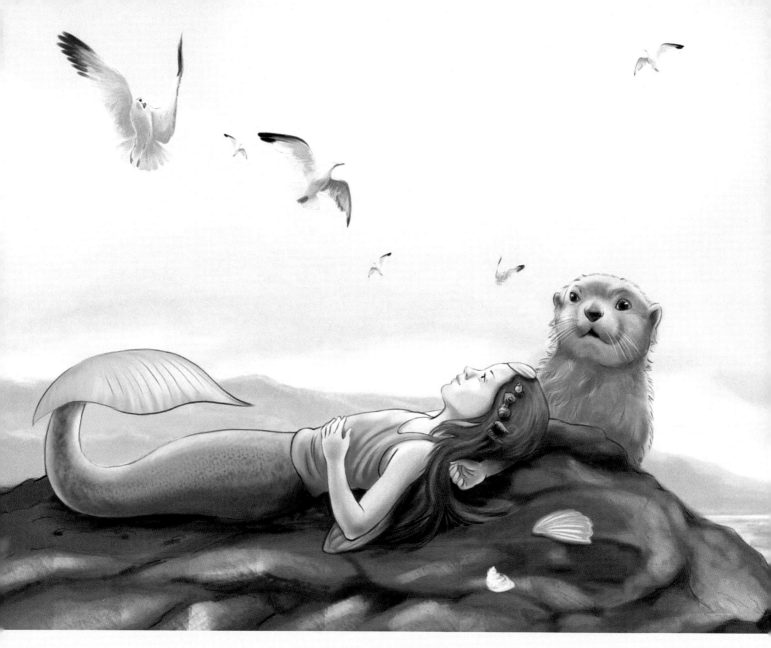

Today he decided to come out from his hiding spot and lie
down right next to the sea child. The sea child was happy
to have company as she watched the seagulls
flying above her head.

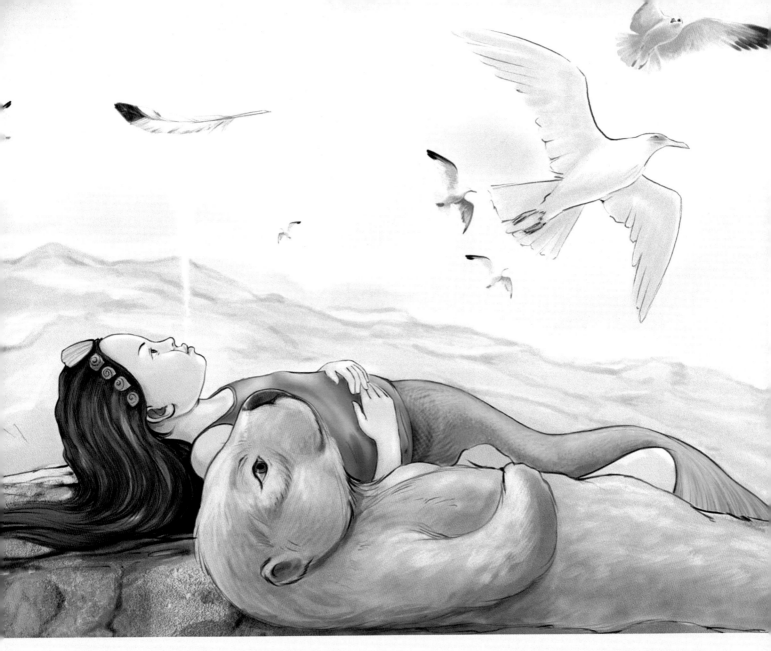

A feather from one of the seagulls circling above her head began to drift down. The sea child laughed as she blew the feather back up towards the clouds. She noticed that when she did this her belly got big and round. She liked the way that this felt. It reminded her of how she used to breathe when she was a baby.

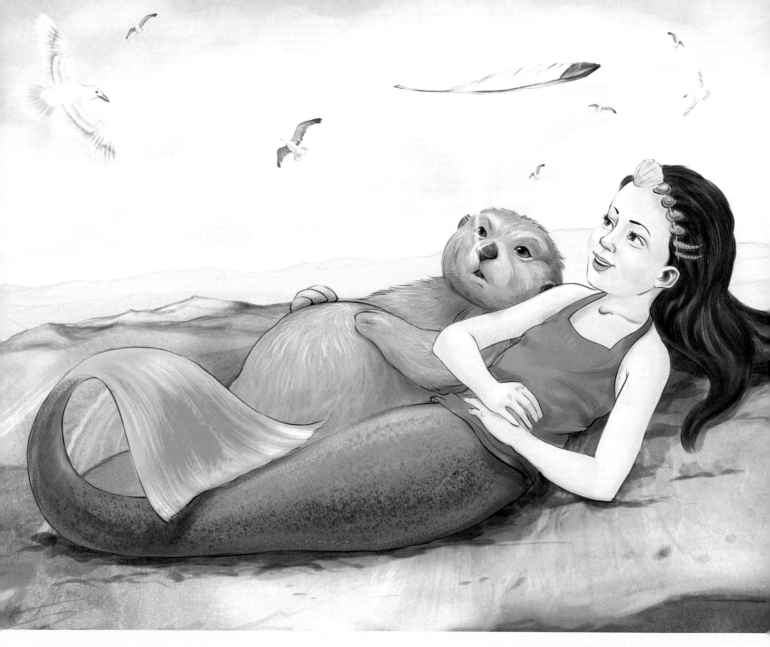

Another feather started to drift down toward her face. The sea child told the sea otter to put his hands on his belly and blow the feather back up towards the clouds. The sea otter blew the feather and felt his belly get big and round. The sea child explained that this is the way his belly should move whenever he practiced healthy breathing.

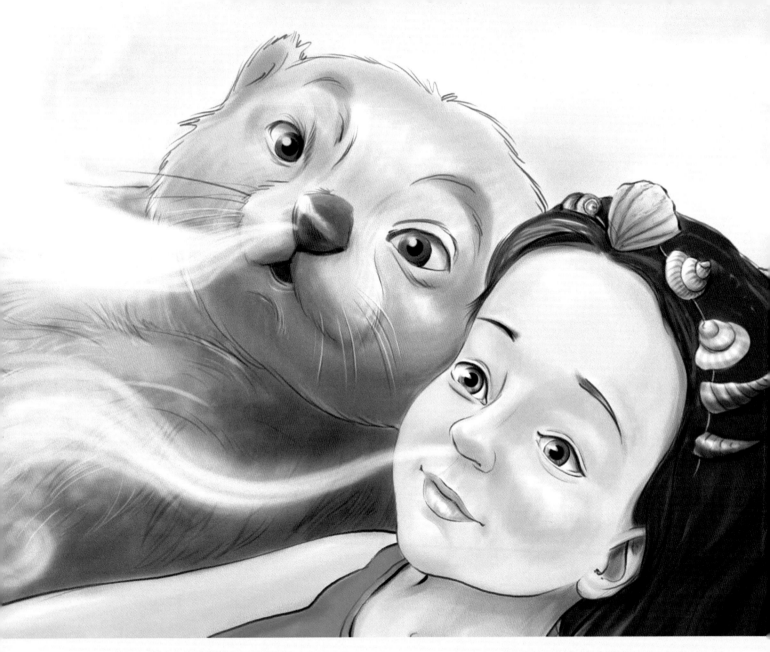

The sea child told the sea otter to breathe in through his nose and out through his nose. He focused all of his attention on the tip of his nose. They both did this breathing together. Breathe in through your nose and out through your nose.

In 2, 3, 4. Out 2, 3, 4...

In 2, 3, 4. Out 2, 3, 4...

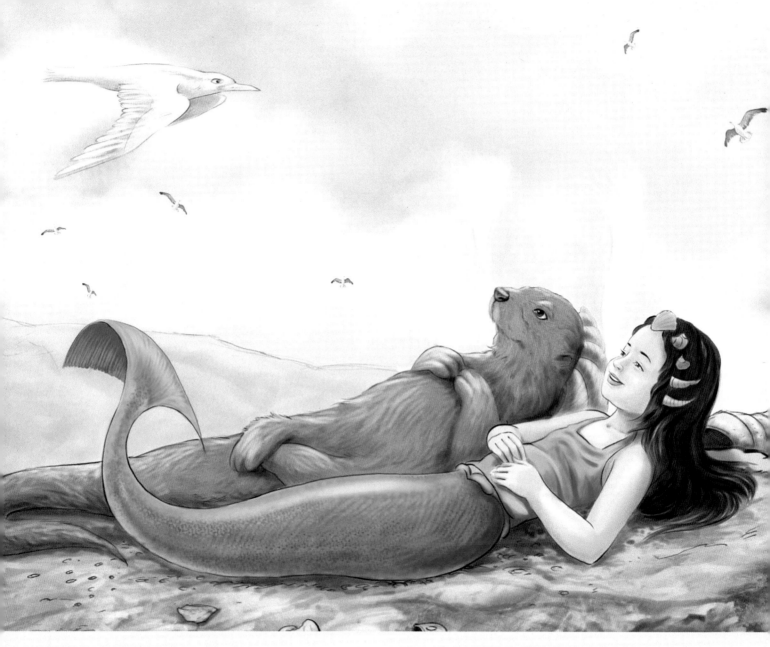

The sea child told the sea otter that he could breathe this way whenever he felt angry or scared or nervous. He could focus on the air moving in and out of the tip of his nose, and he could feel calm and healthy. The sea otter placed his hands on his belly, and felt it lift up and down as the air moved in and out. For a few moments, they both did this breathing together.

Breathe in through your nose and out through your nose.

In 2, 3, 4. Out 2, 3, 4...

In 2, 3, 4. Out 2, 3, 4...

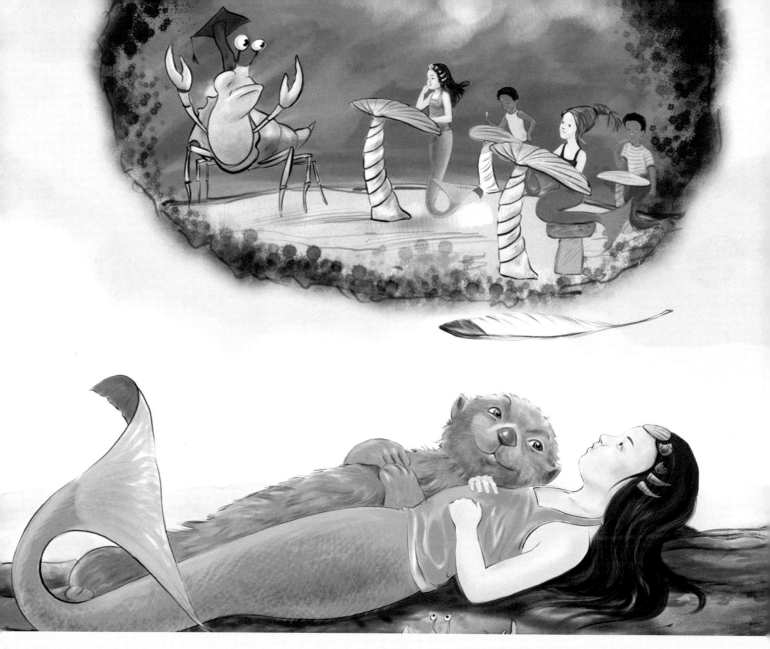

The sea child's mind began to wander. She started thinking about her plans for tomorrow. She imagined that her thoughts were a feather as she blew them away with her next breath out. She focused her attention on her breath again as she drew in a breath of warm fragrant sea air. She liked the way it felt to quiet her mind.

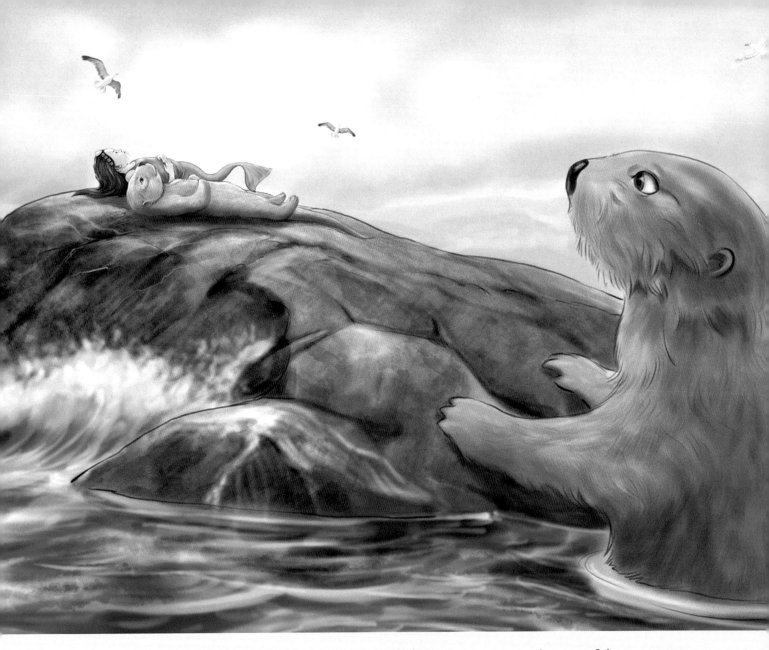

She focused on the way the air felt moving in and out of her nose.
She felt her belly lift up and down as the sea child and the sea otter
continued to breathe together.

Breathe in through your nose and out through your nose.

In 2, 3, 4. Out 2, 3, 4...

In 2, 3, 4. Out 2, 3, 4...

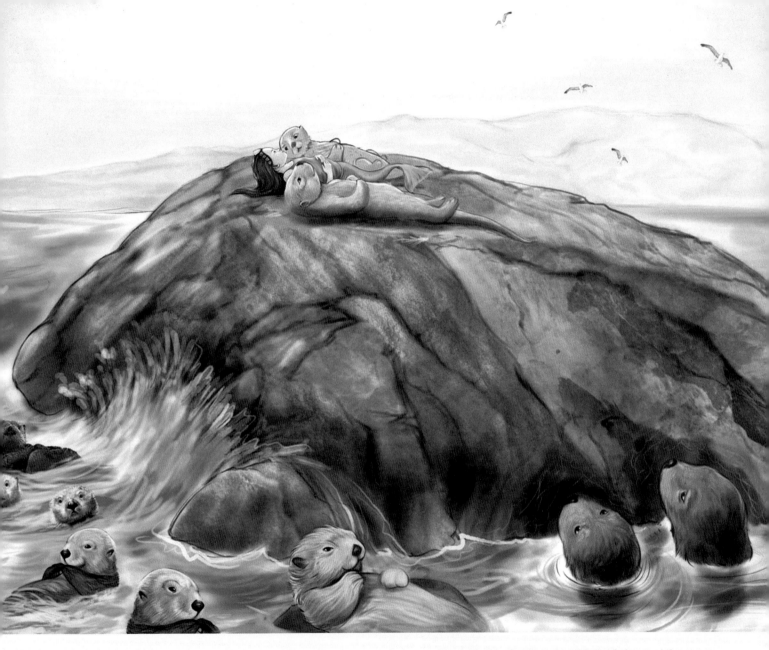

Another sea otter noticed how calm and relaxed the sea child and her friend looked on the rock. She climbed up onto the rock and lay down right next to them.

She began to breathe in through her nose and out through her nose.

In 2, 3, 4. Out 2, 3, 4...

In 2, 3, 4. Out 2, 3, 4...

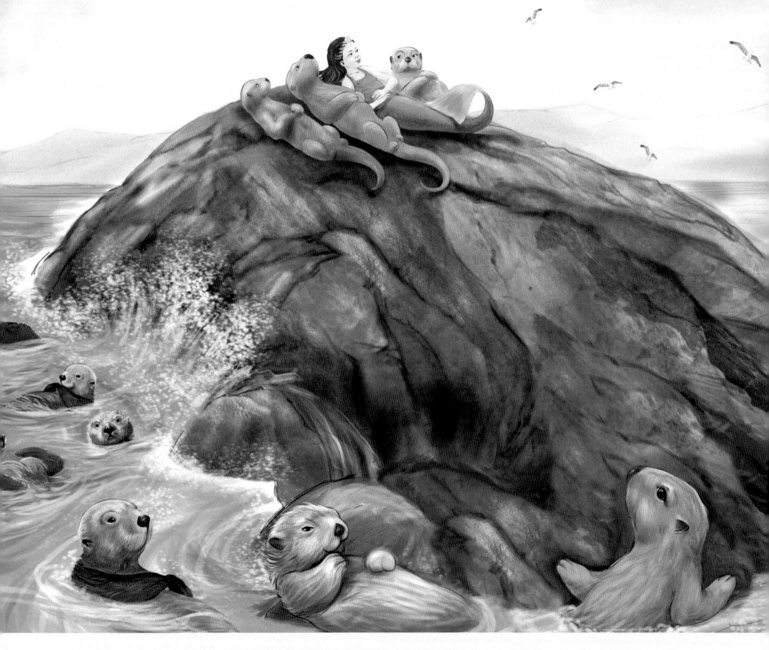

Soon another sea otter playing on the waves noticed how peaceful his friends looked on the rock. He climbed up onto the rock and put his hands on his belly as he joined in with their breathing.

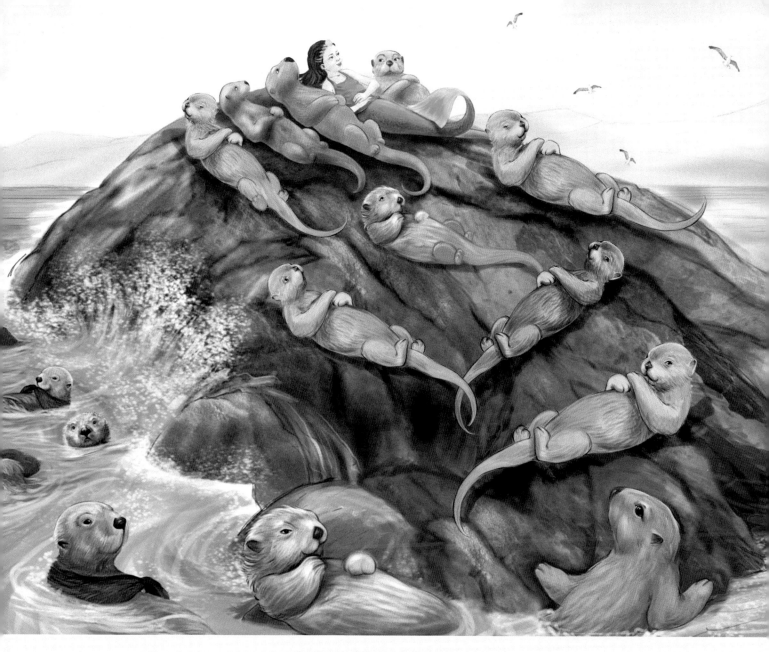

One by one all of the sea otters stopped playing as they too climbed up on the rock. They placed their hands on their bellies and began to breathe in through their nose, and out through their nose.

In 2, 3, 4. Out 2, 3, 4...

In 2, 3, 4. Out 2, 3, 4...

Soon the whole rock was covered with sea otters. They all felt their bellies lift up and down as they joined in breathing with the others.

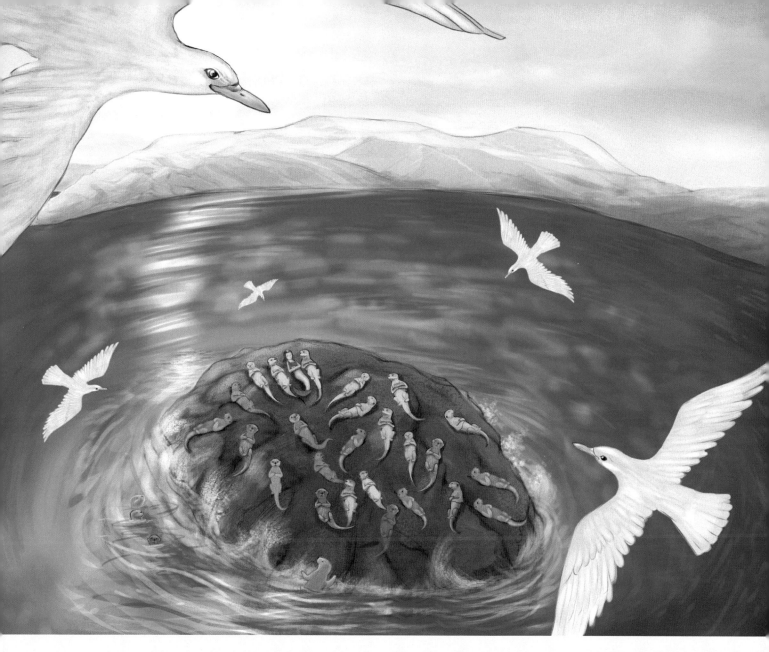

Now the rock was pulsing like a giant heart sending out a pulse of calmness that touched everyone and everything in its path. The breathing pattern was so wonderful and so powerful that it touched the ocean below and the air above.

The seagulls flying above relaxed as they allowed the air to lift them up and down.

Up 2, 3, 4. Down 2, 3, 4...

Up 2, 3, 4. Down 2, 3, 4...

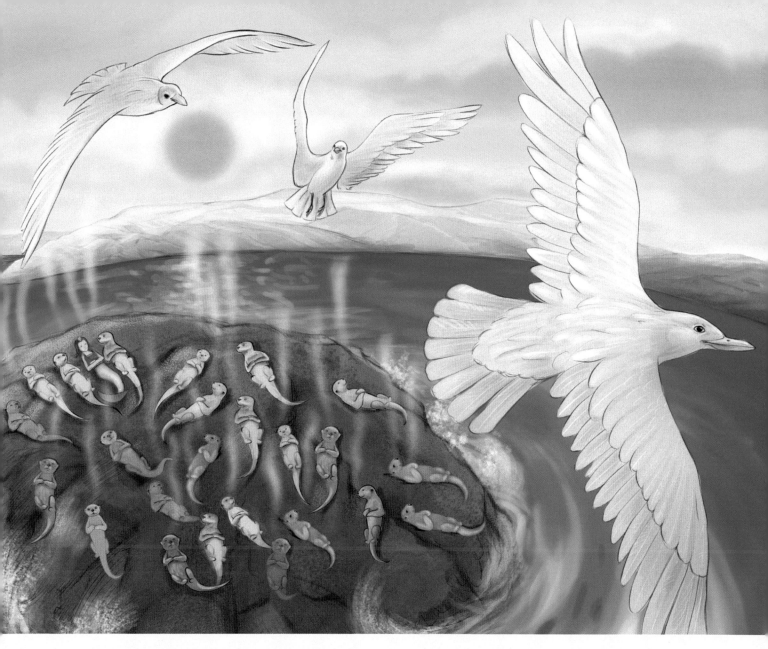

The water was rising and falling as the ocean seemed to sigh.

In 2, 3, 4. Out 2, 3, 4...
In 2, 3, 4. Out 2, 3, 4...
In 2, 3, 4. Out 2, 3, 4...

The rock, the ocean and the seagulls became calmer,

stronger and centered with each breath.

The whole earth was pulsing and breathing in unison.

In 2, 3, 4. Out 2, 3, 4...

In 2, 3, 4. Out 2, 3, 4...

In 2, 3, 4. Out 2, 3, 4...

In 2, 3, 4. Out 2, 3, 4...

Collect the Indigo Dreams Series and watch your whole family manage anxiety, stress and anger…

CD/Audio Books:

Indigo Dreams

Indigo Ocean Dreams

Indigo Teen Dreams

*Indigo Dreams:
Garden of Wellness*

*Indigo Dreams:
Adult Relaxation*

*Indigo Dreams:
3 CD Set*

Music CDs:

*Indigo Dreams:
Kids Relaxation Music*

*Indigo Dreams:
Teen Relaxation Music*

*Indigo Dreams:
Rainforest Relaxation*

Books:

The Goodnight Caterpillar

A Boy and a Turtle

Bubble Riding

Angry Octopus

Sea Otter Cove

Affirmation Weaver

A Boy and a Bear

The Affirmation Web

Resources:

Individual Lesson Plans

Stress Free Kids Curriculum

**Books, CDs and Lesson Plans are available at
www.StressFreeKids.com**

Made in the USA
Columbia, SC
26 September 2020